IT'S EASIER THAN YOU THINK

BY JENNICA MAXFIELD

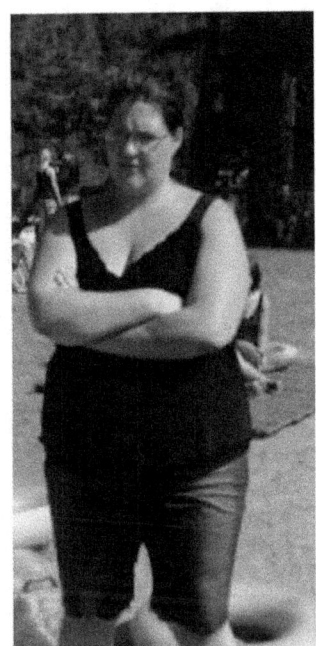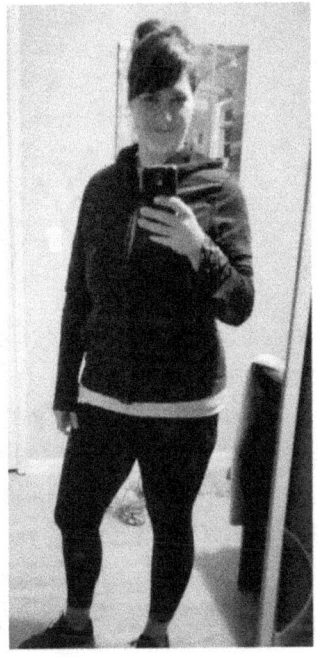

2008 vs 2017 82lbs lost

Intro

This is a quick read. I could have fleshed it out and put in a bunch more personal stories or whatever, but I'm really not into wasting your time or mine. This is not a complicated process and I wanted you to be able to get through it quickly, learn the steps, and get started on your journey asap.

1. My Story

I have always been overweight. As a toddler I was on the chunky side and by the time I was 7 or so, I was quite chubby. I remember being taken to the doctor about my weight when I was 8 years old. It was a horrifically humiliating experience and it was the first time I can remember being aware that I wasn't a 'normal' kid.

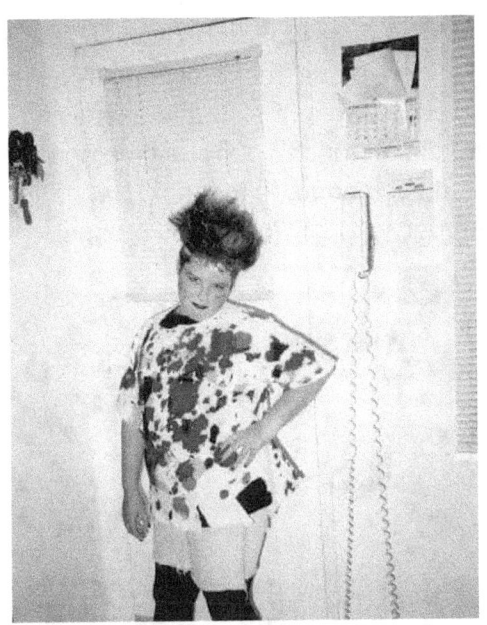

I was about 11 or 12 here

It was shortly after the doctor's visit that I started dieting. Of course, being 8, I didn't have much of a knowledge base for nutrition or what the body needs to function properly. Couple that with the fact that I was a growing girl and you have a recipe for a yo-yo dieting disaster. I spent most of my childhood and teen years on one diet or another. I developed a major addiction to food, using it to deal with boredom, sadness, anger, whatever.

When I was 16, against my better judgement, I signed up for the Miss Princeton pageant. There was a lot of training that went into it as we had to prepare for a fashion show, speech night, and the talent show. Knowing that in four months time I would be standing in front of the entire town really got me motivated to lose weight. I started exercising every night after dinner for an hour at a time and eating very little. It seemed to do the trick. I went from 230 lbs in February of 1997 to 192 lbs by April.

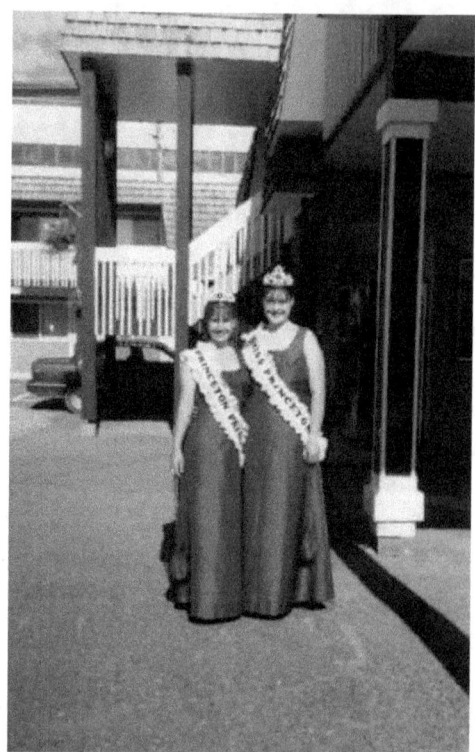

Right around 200 lbs here. It didn't last.

At that point, of course everyone noticed how much weight I had lost and was telling me how amazing I looked. As much as I wanted to keep going and finish losing the weight, I lost momentum at this point. I think having so much positive feedback from people made me feel like maybe I wasn't as fat as I thought I was and that I could take it easier. And as soon as I started taking it easier, the weight starting piling back on. By the time I graduated high school I was back up to 220 lbs.

My upbringing was not exactly conducive to a healthy body image or a healthy lifestyle. I am from the generation of 'clean your plate if you want dessert'. My mom struggled with her weight all her life as well and growing up, I saw a lot of Slim Fast and other fad diets. Diets and weight loss were a constant topic of conversation in our house. We were an incredibly sedentary, unhealthy family as a whole. I saw exercise as a punishment, not as fun. I despised gym class. And because I was so out of shape from lack of regular exercise, I was humiliated every time I had to be active around other kids, unable to keep up. This only perpetuated the cycle of inactivity.

I was extremely fortunate in one respect, though...I can count on one hand the number of times I was ever made fun of for being fat. Even still, being fat became a big part of my identity, a big part of how I defined myself. One of my longest and strongest held beliefs has been that being fat meant a) I was less of a person than other people and b) I was capable of less than other people. I don't know where exactly those beliefs came from, but they have shaped my entire life. It saddens me to think of all the fun and all the opportunities I missed out on because of how I felt about myself as a fat person.

I remember going to summer camp when I was maybe 11 or 12. There was a girl there who was big like me, but unlike me she was loud and outgoing and funny and silly. She spoke her mind, shared her ideas, and wasn't afraid to be the center of attention. She had confidence coming out the ying yang. Everyone loved her. Whenever I had an activity in her group, I would sit there and stare at her in awe. Didn't she know she was fat? Wasn't there some unwritten law about being fat and being required to be shy and awkward and insecure like me??

I spent a large chunk of my adolescence alone. I couldn't handle large groups of people so I always had just one or two friends. I read a lot. I was bored with life and bored with myself. I had no passion for anything and thought the only excitement life held for me was getting the attention of boys. Any boy within a 20 foot radius of me could sense my self-loathing and insecurities and quickly went the other direction. I became so lonely and apathetic that I contemplated suicide.

Nearing graduation I had no idea what to do with my life. I didn't care about anything. I didn't think I was capable of doing anything great. So at the prompting of my dad and my pastor, I enrolled in Bible College. Worst. Decision. Ever. It was even more cliquey than high school and I was there without any friends or family. I borrowed a friend's laptop and spent a LOT of time in chat rooms. It was so easy to be witty and fun when I was hiding behind the keyboard. I had self-confidence to spare.

I met my future husband in one such chat room. When I met him face to face, it was the closest thing to love at first sight I've ever experienced. He was so handsome and I was instantly so much more insecure than ever before. But my weight didn't seem to bother him. In fact, he seemed oblivious to it. We were completely attracted to each other and became inseparable almost immediately. Fast forward a year and we are married with a brand new baby boy.

We were so broke that first year while I was pregnant and what money we did have, we spent irresponsibly, so there wasn't enough money for food a lot of the time. I managed not to put on a bunch of weight with that pregnancy and ended up just 7 lbs heavier than I started. A year and a half after my son was born, I got pregnant with my daughter. This pregnancy was an entirely different story. We were in a slightly better financial position and we were living with my dad, so there was always food. And I ate it. All.

I put on a lot of weight during my second pregnancy and even more after my daughter was born. I ended up around the 250 lb mark, returning to that weight after the births of my third and fourth kids. Fluctuating 5-10 lbs up or down, I kept pretty close to 250 lbs for quite a few years. All the while, of course, I kept trying to diet. I went through Atkins, Body For Life, Slim Fast, starvation, lunch fasting, the Curves program, and a few others I can't remember. All of them were miserable failures.

Then back in 2008, my weight crept up even more and topped out at 282 lbs. I couldn't believe my eyes when I saw that number on the scale. I had no idea when or how or why I had put on so much weight, but I was horrified. I decided that was it, enough was enough, it was time to get the weight off once and for all. I started eating healthier with lots of vegetables and grilled chicken. I walked to and from work, about a 30 minute walk. I went to the gym everyday after work. I worked out every night at home after dinner. My weight refused to budge. I was beyond frustrated.

I hated my body so much. I hated everything about it. I hated the way I looked. I hated the way I felt. I felt hideous and disgusting. I was consumed with thoughts of self-loathing and worthlessness. I felt completely powerless to change and I hated myself for being so weak.

Now I wish I could say I had a defining moment or some great epiphany that spurred incredible weight loss, but I didn't. I started reading a lot of weight loss blogs and books. A lot of them talked about mindful eating and living. I started wondering if I had over complicated this whole weight loss thing. I do have a tendency to overthink and over complicate things, so it wasn't outside the realm of possibility.

The more I thought about it, the more convinced I became that my body was equipped to handle it's own weight loss. I couldn't remember the last time I had eaten according to my body's inborn, biological cues of hunger and satisfaction. I have always eaten because it was 'time' or for emotional reasons, usually as fast as I could. I wondered what might happen if I listened to my body for a change and ate only when I was hungry and stopped when I was full.

And so I began and kept it as simple as that. No exercising. No diets. No calorie counting. No starvation. Just eating mindfully in response to hunger and stopping when I felt satisfied. And lo and behold the weight started to come off! Not super fast, but consistently and immediately. I kept it up and within 6 months was down 30 lbs. I still struggled with self-hatred and extremely low self-esteem, but at least I was starting to lose weight.

As is typical of me, I started to self-destruct when I saw this small bit of success come my way. I plateaued and then gave up. I gained half of the weight back and stayed there until 2013. In March of 2013 I was back on the eat right/exercise bandwagon. I decided to start running. I don't really know why, considering I've always hated running and have tried and failed miserably many times in the past. I think I curious to see if I could change my view of myself in terms of exercise and fitness. I wanted to see if I could set a goal and completely follow through on it.

I got the C25K app for my phone and went to the track 3 times a week to learn how to run. I went turtle slow at first, but I kept at it. After finishing the 9 week program, I was able to run for a full 35 minutes and more than that I found that I loved to run! The healthy eating had fallen by the wayside, but I kept running. Along the way, a few months into my running program, I found my way back to mindful eating. And guess what? The weight started to come off again!

Between April and October of 2013, I lost 50 lbs, bringing my total weight loss to 65 lbs since 2008. In November 2013, my marriage ended. And so did my weight loss. Fortunately it was a very amicable separation so there wasn't any nastiness or bitterness. But still, it was a shock and dealing with that took my focus off of losing weight. During the holidays I ate like I would never see food again, but thankfully because I was still running, I only gained back about 5 lbs.

The next year turned out to be a crazy year for me. Being single as well as having some financial independence for the first time in my adult life, I partied hard and often, made LOTS of questionable choices, and met a lot of *ahem* 'interesting' people. I also started dating and met a guy 22 years older than me in May of 2014. By November we had moved in together and, as often happens to people in relationships after the honeymoon period is over, I started packing on the weight again, eventually landing at 242 lbs.

Somewhat randomly, while looking for something active I could do that might be fun, I joined rugby and fell in love with it. For the first time in my life, my size was a really positive thing. I played as a forward and basically got to bulldoze and destroy anyone who got in my way. It was beyond satisfying and changed how I saw my body. I started to see myself as strong and powerful and began to let go of some of the self-loathing and insecurities that have been with me my whole life.

I didn't lose any weight playing rugby, but it gave me a totally new focus for exercise. Everything physical I did, I did with the intention of getting as strong as possible so I could kick even more ass in rugby. And of course the more I worked out and the stronger I got, the better I felt about my body and the more confident I became. There were also lots of other benefits I reaped as a result like having lots of energy throughout the day, not having excruciating back pain all the time, sleeping like a rock, stuff like that. It was a really exciting time for me.

The two years I spent with that guy were both incredibly amazing and incredibly painful. We were so good together when things were good, which was most of the time. But when things went south, they went hard and fast and big. It was ugly. We finally ended things on Valentine's Day last year (2016).

As difficult as some of our times together were, he did a lot for my self worth over those two years. He helped me to see my value as a person, regardless of my weight, and opened my eyes to the idea that I had a lot of potential and could really do anything I wanted to do in my life. His faith in me helped me to have faith in me. Once I realized that I had no idea what I was truly capable of, I went to work on myself.

I spent a lot of last year really figuring out who I was, who I wanted to be, and what I wanted out this life. I also spent a lot of time challenging myself on how I felt about myself and my body. I read a lot of personal development books and listened to a lot of podcasts. I learned a lot about how powerful our thoughts are in shaping the direction our lives go. And I came to some exciting conclusions.

I realized that I didn't need anyone's permission to go after the things I wanted. And that I deserve, as everyone does, to find happiness and success, whatever those may look like for me. I finally gave myself permission to be great. I finally believed I could be great. And I decided to stop being so damn hard on myself.

Last year was a lot of fun. I saw more change in me in that one year than in all the years before, combined. I faced a ton of fears, saw my way through so many challenges and obstacles, and allowed myself the space to make mistakes and grow from them. My self confidence has exploded...I can't even wrap my head around it sometimes.

I lost about 42 lbs over the last year, again just through intuitive eating, and am sitting at 82 lbs lost overall, and still going. It brought me into 'normal' sizes, which absolutely blows my mind. I've never been able to shop in regular stores before, always plus sized.

I went back and forth for a long time about writing this book for two reasons: I'm not done losing weight...I still have 20 - 30 lbs or so to go. My weight has gone up and down so many times that I wonder how many people would see this method as valid. The conclusion I came to, though,is that I've struggled with this my whole life and I've found a method that is safe and consistent and works when I work at it and I think that's important enough to share with people who are looking for answers.

The other purpose I hope this book serves is to help me finish my weight loss journey. I think that by creating a how-to book of sorts, it will help me to stay on track and remind me of what's missing if I start to falter. It's funny, but when I get in the 'zone' of losing weight, I feel so powerful and invincible and I wonder how I ever struggled before. But when I veer off track, I can't seem to figure out what went wrong or how to get back in line. I want to have this book to refer to in those times.

So thank you for taking the time to read this book. I truly hope you find what you're looking for and that it helps you begin your own journey.

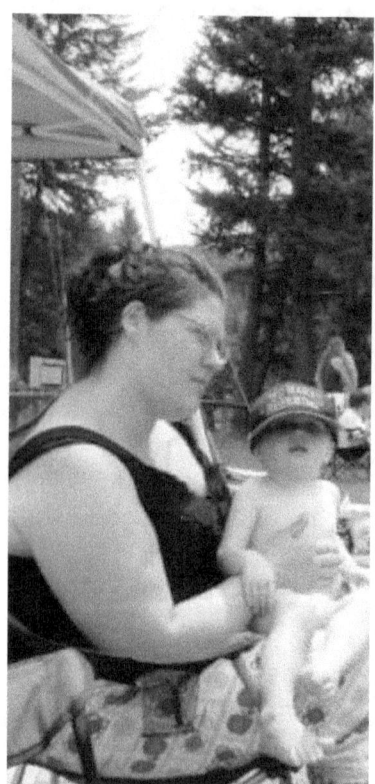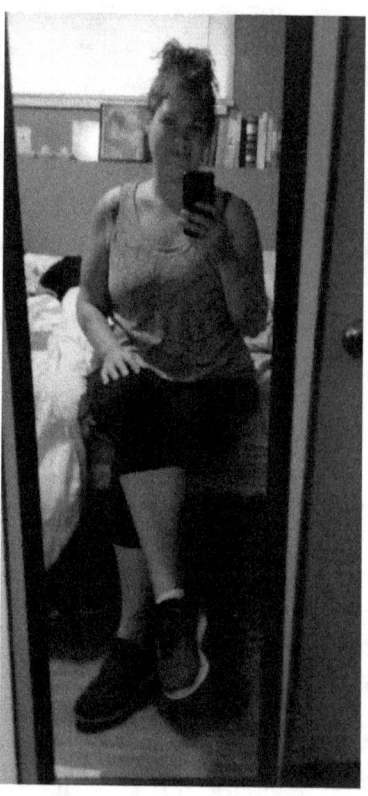

2008 vs 2016 70 lbs lost

2. The Problem

Please keep in mind that I have no medical training or background. What I write here is a summary of my own observations about the struggles so many people face with food and weight loss.

One of the hardest issues I had to deal with regarding weight loss was the sheer number of 'experts' out there touting the latest greatest methods. I have tried so many of them and none of them worked which left me feeling like a complete failure. The trouble is, when I would go through the information on whatever new method I was learning about, it would make sense to me and I could logically see why it would work. So when it didn't, I wondered what might be wrong with me and my body. Which only added fuel to the fire of self-hatred.

Even when I ditched the fad diets and methods and attempted to legitimately eat a balanced, healthy diet and exercise, combining strength training with cardio, I still didn't see any progress. In fact, the last time I tried that, I ended up putting on 10 lbs in a week. Even if that could be explained as muscle or whatever, it doesn't change the fact that the scale was rapidly moving in the opposite direction that I needed it to and I quit. I'm not willing to pour hours and hours of time and pain and sweat into something without seeing any results for weeks or months at a time.

Then there is the question of calories in versus calories out. I tried using those online calculators that take your level of daily activity, height, weight, and age and then tells you how many calories you need in order to lose weight. I have always been way WAY below that number, not an unhealthy amount, mind you, but at least a thousand calories below, yet I still couldn't drop weight. They say a pound of fat is made up of 3500 calories so at the rate I was going, I should have been dropping a pound every few days. No such luck.

I thought maybe I wasn't eating enough, and that my body was unable to let go of the weight, going into starvation mode. So I would increase my calories until I was eating constantly, still not hitting my recommended daily requirements, and I felt sick. And went through groceries like nobody's business. Guess what? My weight went up. ARGH!

Considering how different everyone's bodies are, with different medical histories and different genetic makeups, I question the likelihood of ever being able to calculate exactly what your body requires in order to be healthy AND lose weight at a reasonable rate. Unless you have a medical degree and access to some very expensive technology, I just don't see how this would ever be possible.

What all of these methods never address is the mental and emotional battles that most overweight people have to deal with. It's all well and good to count calories and exercise like a demon, but if you have an addiction to food or eat for any reason other than you're hungry, you're not going to get anywhere. If I hadn't addressed some of the emotional crap that I did, I would never have gained any semblance of control over my eating and lost the weight I did. I still have a lot of junk to handle, but I'm well on my way to being emotionally healthy for the first time in my life.

A big part of the emotional stuff I've had to work on is my perceived reality and my thought patterns. It still amazes me just how much my beliefs about myself and the world around me can help or hinder almost anything I try to do. I use to believe that I was incapable of losing weight, that I didn't deserve to lose weight or be happy, and that I had no control over my eating habits. Those thoughts made it impossible to make any progress. Even if I did well for a little while, the thoughts would pop up and play over and over in my head until I gave in and sabotaged myself.

There was another set of thoughts that went through my head whenever I looked in the mirror too. I hate my belly. I'm so disgusting. I have so much cellulite. My arms look like wings. My ass is huge. And on and on and on. Do you know how hard it is to take care of something you hate? True story. I actually got to the point where I would eat to punish myself for being fat. How messed up is that? I would eat ridiculous amounts of food, knowing full well I would put on weight as a result, all the while telling myself I deserved to be fat and miserable and I could never be anything different.

3. The Solution

Over the last couple of years I have come to find that my body is kind of incredible. All of our bodies are. I think it's in our nature to over complicate and over think things. I know it's in my nature. But it really doesn't have to be complex or confusing or complicated. Our bodies are smart and they are biologically designed to desire the best for themselves. We, of course, treat them like crap and abuse them and take them for granted at which point they start to break down and face problems. But ultimately, our bodies know what weight they should be at and how much food they need to consume to be at that weight. We just stopped listening to them.

The solution is simple. We need to start paying attention again. Our bodies signal us when we are hungry and again when we are full. What I've found in my journey is that my body seems to take into account the extra energy I'm carrying around as fat and adjusts how much fuel it demands in the form of food. I didn't do years of medical research to come to this conclusion. I am making an educated guess here based on my experience with listening to my body's signals and successfully losing weight as a result.

This solution is not about 'good' food versus 'bad' food. It's not about counting calories or eating salad or what you think you 'should' eat. It's about listening to what your body is asking for. In addition to knowing how much energy it needs, your body is also equipped to tell you what it needs in terms of vitamins, minerals, and macronutrients. It communicates these needs to us in the form of cravings. healing your relationship with food and using it only to nourish your body, not to reward, entertain, or soothe yourself.

What I found was that at first, I craved all kinds of crazy crap. Lots of cheese. Chocolate. Greasy food. The worst of the worst. But as I got out of the mindset of 'good' food versus 'bad' food, I found myself craving foods that were actually healthy. When I'm not cramming salad down my throat in the name of weight loss, I actually enjoy salads and other foods that would be classified as 'healthy'. The flip side of that is that I can also enjoy pizza, cake, and burgers when I crave them knowing I am still losing weight.

It really comes down to learning a new approach to food and the way you eat, instead of what you eat. It's about retraining yourself and developing new eating habits. Fairly simple, though not necessarily easy. What I love about it and why it works for me, though, is that it doesn't require special food or supplements, you can start it any time, and you see results almost immediately.

4. The Method

Phase 1

So now that you know the premise of this method, I'm going to break down step by step what I did to lose weight.

The very first thing I should have addressed and that I have to constantly revisit is how I feel about my body. As I said before, and I'm sure you've heard this elsewhere, it's really hard to take good care of and be kind to something you hate. And it's absolutely true. Whenever I've tried approaching weight loss out of disgust for myself, I've been unsuccessful, even when using this method. Just think about that person you loathe. And don't pretend there isn't anyone you can't stand. Everyone's got at least one person that makes them crazy. Now what if I said that I want you to take that person out for a nice meal and then treat them to a spa day? Pretty repulsive thought, no?

The same goes for the way you feel about yourself. If all you do is say awful things to yourself every time you look in the mirror, how likely do you think it is that you'll be successful in taking care of yourself in the form of losing weight? I can tell you from experience that it's almost impossible. I have spent a ridiculous amount of time finding a way to not only accept myself, but to love myself as well.

A great place to start with that was to write down a list of things that are great about me. Accomplishments, personality traits, skills. And while this doesn't really have anything to do with how I feel about my physical body, I found that it is all intertwined. If you love your body, but think you're useless as a human being, you're really not going to get anywhere, are you? After I did that, I spent some time looking in the mirror. Not looking and judging. Not looking and hating. Just looking. I tried to see myself through new eyes, without all of my years of body part specific hatred.

And then I started looking for things I liked about my body. My shoulders. My hair. My feet. My eyes. How well proportioned I am. I made note of all of these attributes and worked on focusing on them rather than the flaws every time I looked in the mirror. Finally, I spent time thinking about all the things my body had done for me. I carried four babies for 9 months each. I nursed each of those babies. I am able to walk. I can also run. I can give and receive hugs. My body has actually done a lot of amazing things for me. Gradually, I started to appreciate and love my body.

Typically, I have enjoyed eating for a lot of reasons other than hunger. I eat for entertainment or when I'm sad or happy. Eating has always been kind of an event for me. I used to love making something uber yummy and sitting down to watch a favourite show on my laptop. Or curling up in bed with a good book and a snack. Or ordering and eating an entire pizza after a rough day. So as well as dealing with my hateful self-talk, I had to deal with what I told myself about food and eating.

I had to reprogram my brain so that I no longer thought of food as entertainment or comfort or an event. Every time I felt the urge to eat for those or any other unhealthy reasons, I would stop and examine how I was feeling and why and then find an alternative that would feed the need. I know a lot of 'experts' have a list of alternatives like 'go for a walk', 'paint your nails', or 'call a friend'. I don't know about you, but when I want to eat, I want to eat and there's no way that going for a walk is going to change that. Nine times out of ten, I end up making some tea with honey or lemon water, just to have something to consume. That one tactic alone has helped me immeasurably in changing my eating habits.

I do want you to be prepared...the mental and emotional stuff is the hardest part of this whole thing. It takes a lot of work and a lot of practice and you may find yourself facing demons you didn't even know existed. It also has a habit of popping up time and time again when you thought you'd dealt with it already. I know for me, there are a lot of different scenarios that can trigger a round of self-directed negative thoughts and emotions. And the worst part is, a lot of the time it's something really minor so it sneaks up on me. Like when I'm all put together in my favourite outfit and feel like I'm looking really good and then I walk past a mirror or store window and I look twice the size I thought I was.

But just because you have to continually revisit this stuff doesn't mean you haven't made progress or that you've failed. You have a lifetime of thought patterns and beliefs to deal with here. They weren't established overnight and they won't be reprogrammed overnight. Keep at it and eventually you won't have to think about it anymore.

Ok so you're dealing with your emotions, thought patterns, and self talk. What's next? Start a journal. Now before you get up in arms about having to get all Dear Diary here, I'm not talking about a second by second account of your every thought/feeling/action (though please feel free if it floats your boat). When I started this process again, I had trouble slowing myself down enough at meal times to think about how I needed to be eating. I would sit down and scarf my meal and when I finished I realized I hadn't come even close to eating mindfully and as a result had eaten too much.

So I started what can loosely be called a journal. Basically, it's a spreadsheet on my laptop where I record the date, what time I'm eating, what I'm eating, and how I'm feeling...whether I'm truly hungry or not and whether I'm feeling in control or rushed or whatever. It forces me to slow down and think about the reasons behind my eating. If I'm eating just for the heck of it, chances are I'm going to reconsider when I have to write it down. It also reminds me what I'm attempting to do. It reminds me that I need to slow down and be mindful throughout the meal.

Aside from the emotional and mental stuff, the biggest part of this whole thing is learning to listen to your body's cues again. It means ignoring the clock and the habits of the people around you and paying attention to what your body is telling you. Forget about the idea that you 'have' to eat breakfast or you'll never lose weight. Forget about 3 square meals a day. Are you hungry? Like legitimately, empty tummy hungry? Then you should eat. Simple as that. Make whatever it is your heart (and body!) desires.

I will offer two warnings here...don't wait until you're absolutely ravenous to make something. If you do and you're anything like me, you will want to eat the quickest, easiest crap you can find. And you're going to wolf it down, forgetting all about mindfulness, worrying only about how fast you can shovel food into your gob. Second, make sure you make a good sized portion of whatever you decide to eat. It should be as much as you would have eaten in full previous to starting this journey. That way, when you eat slowly and mindfully, there will be a bunch left over on your plate when you reach full and you will see how much less you were eating than before.

Alright, you're hungry, you've updated your journal, and made a delicious meal. You are ready to eat. Here's where the magic happens. It's time to retrain yourself in the art of eating. Make sure you have a glass of whatever you feel like drinking. You'll want to sip your drink after every 3 or 4 bites. It helps to slow you down, it helps you digest food better, and it rinses your mouth so you can really taste the food.

As you eat, I would encourage you to chew lots and fully taste the food. Savour every bite. I love to read or watch shows or surf online while I eat (when I'm alone). I know a lot of experts don't recommend this, but here's the logic behind it for me. If I sit down to a meal by myself and have nothing to focus on but the food I get bored. Eating slowly like that takes quite a bit of time and I get bored! Which makes me want to hurry through the meal and defeats the whole purpose. So. I do something while I eat. The difference between this and how I used to eat where food was an event, is that now the activity I choose is the entertainment and the food is just there to fuel me because I'm hungry.

From what I've been told, it takes approximately 20 minutes for your brain to register that you're full. Marking the time I start and stop eating in my journal I can see that it typically takes 15 or so minutes for me to eat and I'm still able to sense that I'm full. Basically when it comes down to it, you should be eating slowly enough that you taste and enjoy each bite and it should take you 15 to 20 minutes to finish.

When you're done, write down the time and how you feel you did in your journal, including whether you were tempted to keep going or content to stop. If you over ate, write that too. Not so you can feel bad about yourself, but so you can have a record of when you struggled and why. You can also use your journal to write about any major or minor events that happen that could trigger emotional eating. When something like that happens for me I like to write down how I did with the trigger, whether I successfully squashed the urge or gave in.

And that's about it! You should start to see the weight coming off after a day or two. Generally I lose a pound every couple of days but everyone is different. As you practice eating this way, make note of how you're feeling physically. If you're someone who is used to eating past the point of full, you're going to feel a lot more comfortable at the end of every meal. I find that the first couple of days are the hardest. What helps, though, is the confidence you start to gain after a few successful meals coupled with the weight starting to come off. It's incredibly encouraging and helps you to keep working at it.

This is not a guaranteed method. I can't promise that it will work for you. As I said before, I am not a doctor or a scientist, nor have I had any formal training. But I have found something that works for me after 33 years of struggling with my weight and if it helps even one person with their weight issues, then I'm happy.

Tips & Tricks

At first you might find, like I did, that you have a hard time pushing your plate away when there's food still on it, especially when it's one of your favourite meals. There are a couple of things you can do to fight the temptation to clean your plate until you've mastered this method.

You may have noticed that food tastes sooooo much better when you're really hungry vs. when you're approaching full. You aren't imagining that...there have been studies done that show that hunger/deprivation can actually increase our sensitivity to flavours. As you get full, that sensitivity decreases[1].

You can use this to your advantage, big time! When you sit down to eat and you're legitimately hungry, instead of approaching your meal from a saving the best for last mentality, flip it around and eat the most delicious looking parts first. By the time you find yourself starting to feel full, all that will be left on your plate is the less desirable, less appetizing leftovers, which are much easier to push away.

Another trick that I used a lot at the beginning, was when there was still food left on my plate and I was tempted to continue eating past the point of satisfied, I would take a bit of water or whatever I was drinking and pour it on the remaining food or put my leftovers away or dump them in the garbage. Then the choice is made for you and you don't have yummy food sitting there staring at you and tempting you.

Something else you can do, that I still do because the benefits are countless, is drink lemon water. All day every day. Besides the fact that it gives you energy, helps your joints and organs function better, and helps flush toxins out of your body, it gives you something to consume that is not empty calories yet still has some flavour and keeps your mouth busy.[2]

Finally, do a bit of mind hacking to overcome the feeling that you're somehow missing out on something when you're leaving food behind. Make it a game to see how much you can leave on your plate while still feeling full. Get excited to see all that food still sitting there and realize that you don't feel deprived. And if something is ridiculously delicious and you just can't come to terms with not getting to eat all of it, save it for later! I've had leftovers from restaurants last me 3 meals this way. Getting to enjoy your favourites over and over is incredibly rewarding!

Phase 2

So here's where I'm at now. Phase 2...mostly. I still have my struggles with overeating sometimes and from time to time will find myself falling into old habits, but for the most part, intuitive eating is pretty much second nature to me. I still have between 20 to

30 lbs to go, though I'm far less interested in the scale these days, knowing it'll come off as I maintain this lifestyle.

Phase 2 is an exciting place to be. I've dropped enough weight now that for the first time in my life I can shop in non plus sized stores. I can wear shorts and sleeveless shirts and dresses without feeling self-conscious. I can walk up stairs without getting winded. I feel comfortable in my own skin.

Losing this weight has been the most incredible journey of my life. For anyone who has struggled with their weight for any significant amount of time, you know how all-consuming it can be. From the way you feel about your body, to obsessing about food, to the constant search for a solution, it sucks up so much of your energy and focus. It's exhausting and depressing.

Gaining control over and freedom from the eating compulsions that have plagued me since I was young is something I never thought possible for me and has radically transformed my life and the way I see myself. Aside from the weight loss itself, this success has given me such a profound sense of personal power and accomplishment. It has given me the confidence to pursue so many other great big goals in a bunch of areas that I would never have considered for myself before.

That's kind of what Phase 2 is all about. It begins when you no longer view yourself as 'fat'...when the vocabulary you use to describe yourself is full of words of positivity and self-love, focusing on who you are at your core instead of what you look like. It starts when you can look in the mirror and appreciate what you see, top to bottom. It also starts when you can approach food and eating with a sense of peace and joy, having overcome the helpless mindset that used to tell you that you had no self control.

I mean, theoretically you could just go through Phase 1 and lose the weight and continue eating all the foods you've always loved and leave it at that. But I feel that I would be doing you a disservice if I said that was as good as it gets and that's where your journey ends. You can actually take it one step further and feel the best you've ever felt in your life. That's Phase 2.

This is where it gets really fun. You get to take all that focus and energy that you used to waste on food and weight related garbage, and put it onto taking the best care of your body and mind that you possibly can. Once you have stopped looking at food as either bad or good, you can start to look at it in terms of what the most nourishing and beneficial food is that you can put into your body.

There is so much good food out there that is nutritionally dense, which is exciting because It opens up a new world of possibilities in the realm of meal options. You might be surprised, as I was, at how much your tastes change over time when you eat intuitively.

Since I gave up trying to eat 'healthy' when I started this process and learned that I could eat all the crap food I've always loved AND lose weight at the same time, I did just that. I ate nothing but crap and wouldn't touch vegetables of any kind with a 10 foot pole. It was such a thrill to go to McDonalds and order whatever I wanted, knowing I could eat it and still lose weight. It actually took me a long time to fully wrap my head around that.

When I finally got over the novelty of that whole concept, I started to notice that all this garbage food I was craving and eating was not really satisfying me anymore or tasting quite so good. In fact I was shocked to find some of these previously delicious indulgences to be kinda...bland and gross. What the hell? I also found that I didn't much like the way I felt when I ate these foods.

After a lot of meals I often felt heavy, tired, and lethargic. And seeing as how I had started to be more active with rugby and running and working out, I needed as much energy as possible in order to perform at my best. There's nothing worse than trying to run at top speed with a belly full of processed, fatty foods. Blech.

I also started to learn more about the effects of sugar, bad fats, and processed foods on the body. That's some scary stuff, man. Cancer, arthritis, inflammation, early aging, Alzheimer's, heart disease, diabetes, and so on and so on and so on. When you've made peace with your body and actually love it and want to take care of it, it's pretty tough to reconcile those food choices with this new self love frame of mind. They just don't line up.

That doesn't mean, however, that you never touch sugar again. Or give up pizza. Or even that you completely overhaul your pantry and fridge in one day, getting rid of all your favourite foods. But in the spirit of intuitive eating and mindfulness, start to pay attention to how you feel when you eat and what foods make you feel really good and what foods don't. Consider, when you're figuring out what to eat, how nourishing you want your meal to be. The foods you eat have incredible power. They can poison you, drain you, and make you sick. Or they can heal you, energize you, and help your body to work exactly as it's supposed to.

Nutritious, wholesome food doesn't have equate to boring, rabbit food. I've found a ton of recipes that are infinitely more flavourful and satisfying than any of my old nutritionally bankrupt favourites. As a bonus, I've included a bunch of them for you at the end of the book. You're welcome!

The cool thing is, once you start introducing good for your body foods into your rotation of regularly consumed grub, you are reprogramming your gut bacteria to actually crave more of the nutritious stuff and less of the stuff that only pleases your taste buds[3]. It's a pretty kickass cycle.

Before you know it, you'll accidentally on purpose be living the 80/20 lifestyle, which basically means that 80% of the time you eat clean, whole foods that nourish your body and 20% of the time you are free to indulge, guilt free in any food that floats your boat. The point of Phase 2 is to find balance, to find a way of living that you can maintain for the rest of your life.

By now you should have the tools you need to get moving on your weight loss journey. Don't get too hung up on 'rules' here. The most important step in all of this is getting to know yourself and why you do the things you do. Sometimes that means trying different things and making modifications as you go.

[1] BioMed Central. "Food Tastes Stronger When You're Hungry." ScienceDaily. ScienceDaily, 23 February 2004. Web. 26 Mar, 2017.
[2] Joe Leech, Dietitian. "Lemon Water 101: What Are The Benefits Of Drinking It?". *Authority Nutrition*. N.p., 2017. Web. 26 Mar. 2017.
[3] Ho, Vincent. "How the bacteria in our gut affect our cravings for food." The Conversation. N.p., 16 Mar. 2017. Web. 26 Mar. 2017.

5. P.S.

Please don't skimp on the mental work of changing how you feel about yourself, your body, and food. I think this is why I lost and gained so many times...I didn't take the time to truly address these issues. Your mind is so freaking powerful. If you have a cycle of crappy thoughts running in your subconscious all the time, your actions are going to follow whether you want them to or not.

If you don't know where to start, here is a mini workbook with some actions you can take to start disrupting and reprogramming your old thought patterns. Some of them may seem ridiculous, and they are. But they work. If you want to get different results than you've been getting, you're going to have start doing things differently. It's worth it, I promise! Do this at your own speed, take your time on each one, there is no rush. The point is build new habits, one on top of the other, not to massively makeover your whole life in one sitting.

- Fill in the first column where with statements about your current beliefs regarding food, exercise, yourself, and your body. In the second, create new statements, healthy statements. I've added some examples to start you off.

I eat when I'm bored or angry or sad or happy.	I listen to my body and eat only when I'm hungry.
I hate my body, it's fat and disgusting	I'm thankful for my body, it's strong and carries me through each day
I hate exercise	Moving my body feels good and I love taking care of myself
I can't lose weight, I'll always be fat	If I listen to my body and take care of it, the weight will come off.

Now take your new truths and put them on sticky notes or index cards and keep them close by. Repeat them to yourself throughout the day. Every time you notice a garbage thought popping up, interrupt it with your new belief. Look yourself in the eye in the mirror when you say them. I guarantee you'll feel like a knob, but it will help make them stick. You won't believe them at first. But remember that you're working against thoughts and beliefs that have been in place for years. Be relentless. Keep at it until you believe these new patterns.

- Write down your why's. Why do you want to lose weight? What will that mean in your life? Write down as many as possible. You want to create a tangible, compelling list of reasons to stay on track in your weight loss journey so that when you feel discouraged and tired, you can refer to it and be reminded of why you started in the first place.

  1. _____
  2. _____
  3. _____

4. _____

5. _____

6. _____

7. _____

8. _____

9. _____

10. _____

11. _____

12. _____

13. _____

14. _____

15. _____

16. _____

17. _____

18. _____

19. _____

20. _____

- Start practicing gratitude. All day every day. I'm not trying to turn you into Polly Positive here, but the simple fact is that it's really hard to be negative and focus on negative stuff when you're actively grateful. Try it, I dare ya. And the more you focus on the good stuff in your life, the better you'll feel and the more good stuff will come your way. And your body will respond big time to you feeling good!

Take a minute and think of 10 things you are grateful for today:

1. _____
2. _____
3. _____
4. _____
5. _____
6. _____
7. _____
8. _____
9. _____
10. _____

Reflect on this list often. Add to it often.

- Know your struggles and triggers and plan ahead for them. Willpower and white knuckling your way through temptations is not a plan. It's a nice concept and works sometimes, but as an ongoing course of action not so much. Remember that you're fighting against some really powerful, likely long time struggles here. You have to be proactive and create a battle plan.

If you know that you get the munchies every night when you sit down to watch your favourite show, you can't expect to just ignore it and hope it goes away. In that particular scenario, as soon as the urge to munch hits you, grab a cup of tea or a lemon water and go over your new statements from the first exercise. Remind yourself that food does NOT control you, you control it. Also go over the list of why you want to lose weight. Stand in front of the mirror and look yourself in the eye while you say it out loud to yourself. Yea yea, I know it sounds stupid. But ask yourself this...would you rather feel silly for a while, but overcome this whole food/weight thing, or do what you're comfortable with and used to and forever be a slave to food?

Use the space below to write down your triggers. Anything you can think of. TV is a huge trigger for a lot of people. Think about your emotional triggers as well like having a garbage day and craving a binge night of comfort foods. Beside each trigger, write down your plan to kick the crap out of it.

Trigger	Plan of Action

The trick here is to actually put these plans into action. Immediately. No humming and hawing about what to do when you find yourself facing temptation. Research says we have about 5 seconds to take action when we have the impulse to do something new before your brain defaults to old, learned behaviors. Mel Robbins actually wrote a book called The

5 Second Rule (https://melrobbins.com/the-5-second-rule/) based on this research. I would encourage you to read up on it and implement it. It's incredibly powerful.

- Start moving your body. Please note, I did not say go sign up at the gym and spend six hours a day working out and sweating your ass off. What I'm saying is find something you can do to move your body that feels good and will start releasing those endorphins. Dance in your living room for 15 minutes. Call a friend and go for a walk. Do some yoga. Whatever. The point is to stop looking at exercise as a torturous activity you have to do if you want to lose weight. And bonus points if you can actually find something fun to do. Play, explore, see what feels good. Your body is amazing and will surprise you with what it can do when you take the time to take care of it. If you can move the focus of exercise off of weight loss and give yourself an unrelated goal, you are much more likely to stick with it. When I started running, the goal was to be able to run longer than 6 minutes, which was the longest I had ever run when I was in high school. The more I practiced running, the more I enjoyed it and how it made me feel. Eventually, I started to see myself as a runner. Which in turn changed so much about how I felt about my body. Ditto with rugby. I became an athlete, not just a fat girl who was trying out a sport.

In the space below, write down a fitness goal you would like to start working towards and a plan of action to get there. Whether it's going for a 30 minute walk every day or running a 5k, find something you can do, not to lose weight, but to feel good in your body.

Fitness goal:

_____

_____

Plan of action:

_____

_____

_____

_____

- Buy and eat the best food you can afford. Stop looking at it in terms of 'good' and 'bad'. Approach food with the desire to nourish and take care of your amazing body. Go for flavour and delicious texture and substance. Eat food that you love, not just food that is easy. Explore new dishes and flavours.

Choose a new recipe to try today and jot down some quick notes about your experience with it.

_____

_____

_____

_____

_____

_____

- Get enough sleep. I cannot stress this enough. When you are constantly tired, you don't have the energy or desire to make good choices for yourself regarding these new habits you're trying to build. You go with what's easiest and slip back into old behaviors and thought patterns.

  According to Scientific American[1], our brains gobble up to 20% of our daily energy supply. If your energy supply is crazy low because you're not getting enough sleep, your brain is is not going to be firing on all cylinders and when it's faced with the choice between expending energy to implement new behaviors and going with what's easy and familiar, I'll give you three guesses what it's going to go with.

- Get connected. Partner up with someone. Join a Facebook group. Find a Meetup. It is so so so important to have people in your life to support you as you go after what you want. Especially when you falter or feel like giving up. They will keep you accountable and remind you what a badass you are when you need it most. On the flip side, offering accountability to someone else will serve to strengthen your commitment to this whole process. When you know someone is counting on you to hold them accountable, it puts you in something of a leadership position and drives you to be a good example.

I will be accountable to _____ starting on , 20___.

I will check in once a day/week via

_____(Facebook, email,

phone, face to face meeting)

- Personal development. I cannot say enough about this, not just from a weight loss standpoint, but from a life standpoint. Work on yourself, every day. Read books, listen to podcasts, go to events. You have more potential than you could ever imagine. Don't you want to become that absolute best version of yourself possible? You are so worth the investment. Personal development is such an addictive process. You learn so much about yourself, you discover new passions and interests, you open up a whole new world of possibilities for yourself.

Today I listened to/read

_____

I learned

_____

_____

_____

_____

- And speaking of investing in yourself...treat yourself from time to time. Get a massage, take a relaxing bath, get a haircut, buy a new outfit. You are a worthwhile person, you have huge value, and you deserve to have and do nice things. Communicate this to your mind and body as often as you can.

Write down 5 things you can do to treat yourself that would make you feel good about you:

    1. _____

       _____

2. _____

_____

3. _____

_____

4. _____

_____

5. _____

_____

_____

Now pick one of those and DO IT! Like today. Like now.

- STOP COMPARING YOURSELF TO OTHER PEOPLE!!! Did you hear me? Knock it off! You are you...your journey, your past, your experiences, they are all unique to you. You don't know where other people have come from or where they're going and it really doesn't have any bearing on you at all. I finally got this through my thick skull a few months ago. It was a huge AHA! moment, let me tell you. I was chatting with a friend of mine, this amazing, successful, kind, gorgeous, accomplished, kickass woman. We were talking about our challenges and struggles and she basically said she felt she was just meh. Like she didn't recognize how incredible she was and how many people thought the world of her and wanted to be just like her. She felt there were so many other women out there who were better than her and that she had a long way to go to really feel 'successful'. I thought, holy crap! If a woman like that could feel that way about herself after everything she's done, what hope do I have? I made a decision that day that I was never again going to compare myself to anyone else. The bottom line is, everyone has insecurities, everyone has stuff about them they wish they could change. I just want to be the best me. I'm going to celebrate the crap out of my victories and learn from my failures and just keep working. End of story.

List 5 things about you that you love, physical or otherwise:

1. _____

2. _____

3. _____

4. _____

5. _____

_____

Now the next time you find yourself look at someone else and lamenting how much prettier/smarter/more accomplished they are than you, remind yourself that you don't know their story or their struggles and come back to this list. You need to be your number one fan. It is not arrogance, I promise. You need to be able to stand firm in the knowledge of your awesomeness.

- For the love of all that is holy, please allow yourself the time to get where you want to go. I totally get that you would give your firstborn to fast track to the end of the process and have the weight gone. But I wasted 32 or so years looking for a way to fast track. It doesn't exist and I could have gotten there years ago if I had stopped looking for a quick fix. Please learn from my mistakes. The time is going to pass anyways. Enjoy the journey, know that it will be so so worth it, and do the work.

- Document your successes. Weight related and otherwise. Our brains have a tendency to focus on the negative. If you have a day where you struggle with meals and overeat or eat when you're not hungry or if the scale doesn't move for a couple of days, it could be easy to get down on yourself and fall back into old habits and old ways of thinking. Writing down your victories will serve as an excellent reminder of what you're capable of. One bad meal or one bad day doesn't mean failure. Learn from it, correct your behaviour, and keep moving forward.

Write down 3 things you kicked ass at today (doesn't matter how big or small):

1. _____

2. _____

3. _____

_____

- Create new rewards for yourself outside of food. Building on the last step regarding celebrating your successes, you need to find ways to reward yourself proportionately for those successes. For example, when I was just getting started with running, I decided that if I stuck with my running program to the end, which was 9 weeks, I would buy myself my first EVER brand new pair of name brand running shoes. Let me tell you, as someone who doesn't spend money on herself often and is used to second hand everything, this was an awesome goal to work towards for me and it kept me motivated and accountable. I rocked that running program and I got those shoes and it felt amazing!

Keep in mind, though, it doesn't necessarily have to be something huge like that. The idea is to positively reinforce these new habits you're building and to celebrate ALL of your victories, big and small, in some way. This is a good time to refer back to the list you made of things you can do to treat yourself. If you are someone who has a hard time doing nice things for yourself just because, this is an excellent opportunity for you. You can treat yourself guilt free because you freaking earned it

List 5 ways you are going to reward yourself for your weight loss and non-scale victories:

1. _____

   _____

2. _____

   _____

3. _____

   _____

4. _____

   _____

5. _____

   _____

[1]Swaminathan, Nikhil. "Why Does the Brain Need So Much Power?" Scientific American. Scientific American, a Division of Nature America, Inc., 29 Apr. 2008. Web. 26 Mar. 2017.

6. Personal Development

If you're taking my advice to heart about how important personal development is, here's a list of some of my favourite books and podcasts as a jumping off point:

Books:
- You are a Badass by Jen Sincero
- Choose Yourself by James Altucher
- Success Principles by Jack Canfield
- Awaken the Giant Within by Tony Robbins
- Big Magic by Elizabeth Gilbert
- The Four Agreements by Don Miguel Ruiz
- Love Yourself Like Your Life Depends on It by Kamal Ravikant
- The Monk Who Sold His Ferrari by Robin Sharma

Podcasts:
- Earn Your Happy - Lori Harder
- The James Altucher Show
- Good Life Project - Jonathan Fields
- The Art of Charm - Jordan Harbinger
- Happier - Gretchen Rubin
- The School of Greatness - Lewis Howes

- Pivot - Jenny Blake

So what are you waiting for?? You have the tools to get started. Forget Monday, start with your next meal. You can do this, you deserve this, now go make it happen!

7. Recipes!

As promised, here are some of my favourite whole foods recipes.

Portobello Benedict

Author: Kari Lund

Ok, this is seriously one of my all time favourite brekkie recipes. This hollandaise sauce is TO DIE FOR. And you'll notice...butter, oh so much butter. And bacon. YUM! But also spinach, and mushrooms. The combination is delicious!

Yield: Serves 1

Ingredients:

- 1 portobello mushroom cap
- 1 egg
- 2 slices Canadian bacon
- Handful of fresh spinach leaves
- Chives and fresh ground pepper for garnish
- Hollandaise sauce (optional)

For the Hollandaise:

- 2 egg yolks
- 1/4 teaspoon Dijon mustard
- 1 teaspoon lemon juice
- 4 Tablespoons melted butter
- 1/8 teaspoon salt
- Pinch of cayenne pepper

Method:

1. Preheat oven to 350 degrees Fahrenheit.
2. In a muffin tin, add 1 tablespoon water and egg. Bake 8-10 minutes. Lift egg out with a slotted spoon and dry gently on a clean kitchen towel.
3. While egg is baking, heat a sauté pan with olive oil on medium heat.
4. Add portobello mushroom cap and Canadian bacon. Sauté until bacon is lightly browned and mushroom is slightly soft.
5. To assemble, place spinach on plate, then mushroom cap, Canadian bacon, egg, and top with hollandaise, chives, and pepper.

For the Hollandaise:

1. Combine all hollandaise ingredients in a small saucepan and cook over low heat until thickened, whisking constantly, for about 5 minutes.

https://breakingmuscle.com/fuel/mushrooms-in-the-morning-portobello-benedict

Chocolate Coconut Granola

Author: MOMables.com

Ok, so chocolate anything for breakfast? Nuff said.

Yield: 7 Cups

Ingredients

- 4 cups rolled oats
- 1 cup shredded coconut
- ½ cup flaxseeds
- 1 cup chopped nuts or shelled seeds (optional)
- ½ cup cocoa powder
- ⅓ cup melted coconut oil
- ½ teaspoon vanilla extract
- ⅓ cup maple syrup
- ¼ cup brown sugar
- ¼ cup mini chocolate chips

Instructions

1. Preheat the oven to 325F. Grease a large baking sheet with a little coconut oil.
2. In a large bowl, stir together the oats, coconut, flaxseeds, and nuts (if using).
3. In a medium bowl, whisk together the cocoa, oil, vanilla, maple syrup, and brown sugar until smooth. Pour the chocolate mixture over

the oat mixture in the large bowl, and stir until all the oats are coated.

4. Distribute the mixture evenly into the bottom of the prepared baking sheet, and bake for 15 minutes. 5. Remove from the oven, then stir, and bake for another 15 minutes.

5. Remove from the oven again, and allow the granola to cool completely in the pan without stirring.

6. Once it's cooled completely, add in the mini chocolate chips. Store in an airtight container.

http://www.momables.com/chocolate-coconut-granol a-recipe/

Red Curry Lentils
Author: Pinch of Yum

This is by far my favourite meatless dinner. My kids even like it. So much flavour, so filling, a bit of spice. So good!

Yield: serves 6

Ingredients

- 1½ cups lentils, rinsed and picked over
- ½ large onion, diced
- 2 tablespoons butter
- 2 tablespoons red curry paste
- ½ tablespoon garam masala
- 1 teaspoon curry powder
- ½ teaspoon turmeric
- 1 teaspoon sugar
- 1 teaspoon minced garlic
- 1 teaspoon minced ginger
- a few good shakes of cayenne pepper
- 1 14 ounce can tomato puree
- ¼ cup coconut milk or cream
- cilantro for garnishing
- rice for serving

Instructions

1. Cook the lentils according to directions. Drain and set aside.

2. Melt the butter in a large saucepan over medium high heat. Add the onion and saute for a few minutes until fragrant and golden. Add all the spices (curry paste, garam masala, curry powder, turmeric, cayenne, sugar, garlic, ginger) and stir fry for 1-2 minutes. Add the tomato puree; stir and simmer until smooth.
3. Add the lentils and the cream. Stir to combine and simmer for another 15-20 minutes (the longer, the better)! Serve over rice and garnish with cilantro.

http://pinchofyum.com/red-curry-lentils

Homemade Mushroom Soup
Author: Season with Spice

This soup makes my soul happy. It is so rich and mouthwateringly flavourful.

Serves 2 as appetizer

Ingredients:
300g or 2 cups fresh mushrooms - cleaned and chopped finely
1 tbsp olive oil
3-4 cloves garlic - chopped
1 tbsp butter
1/2 tbsp chopped fresh thyme or 1/4-1/2 teaspoon of dried thyme (optional)
1 bay leaf
2 tsp Worcestershire sauce
1 cup chicken or vegetable stock
1 tbsp flour dissolved in 1 tbsp water
Salt to taste
1/2 cup heavy cream
1/2 cup milk
Dash of nutmeg
Freshly ground black pepper to taste
Fresh parsley or thyme for garnish

Method:
1. Heat olive oil in a sauce pan. Add butter and lightly sauté garlic on medium heat.
2. Add in mushrooms, thyme, bay leaf, and Worcestershire sauce. Cook over medium heat for 5

minutes, or until the moisture from the mushrooms disappears.

3. Add in chicken broth. Stir occasionally until broth boils, then reduce heat and simmer for 10 minutes.

4 Add diluted flour in, and stir constantly (while simmering) until the mixture thickens. Season with salt and nutmeg. Taste and adjust seasonings.

5. Finally, add milk and heavy cream, and bring to a simmer. Turn heat off.

6. Transfer to soup bowls. Add freshly ground black pepper. Garnish with fresh parsley or thyme if you have them on hand.

Turkey Burgers with Zucchini

Author: skinnytaste.com

Throw a little chipotle mayo on top, maybe some Monterey Jack cheese....aw yea!

Yield: 5 burgers

Ingredients

- 5 oz grated zucchini (when squeezed 4.25 oz)
- 1 lb 93% lean ground turkey
- 1/4 cup seasoned whole wheat breadcrumbs*
- 1 clove garlic, grated
- 1 tbsp grated red onion
- 1 tsp kosher salt and fresh pepper
- oil spray

Directions:

1. Squeeze ALL the moisture from the zucchini with paper towels.
2. In a large bowl, combine ground turkey, zucchini, bread crumbs, garlic, onion, salt and pepper.
3. Make 5 equal patties, 4 1/2 ounces each, not too thick so they cook in the center.
4. Heat a large nonstick skillet on high heat. When hot, lightly spray oil.

5. Add burgers to the pan and reduce the heat to low. Cook on one side until browned, then flip.
6. Flip over a few times to prevent burning and to make sure the burgers are cooked all the way through.

http://www.skinnytaste.com/turkey-burgers-with-zucchini/

Apple Pecan Feta Spinach Salad

Author: cookingclassy.com

I love this salad because it's got substance! Between the bacon and the feta and the cranberries and the pecans, it's super filling and ridiculously delicious!

Yield: About 7 - 8 servings

Ingredients

- 10 oz baby spinach
- 3 small gala apples or 2 medium, cored and thinly sliced
- 1 cup pecans, toasted
- 4 oz feta cheese, crumbled (don't use the pre-crumbled stuff)
- 1/2 cup dried cranberries
- 12 oz bacon, cooked and crumbled (optional)
- 1/2 small red onion, sliced into thin strips (optional)

Maple-Cider Vinaigrette

- 1/2 cup olive oil
- 1/4 cup apple cider vinegar
- 2 Tbsp pure maple syrup
- 2 tsp dijon mustard
- 1/4 tsp salt
- 1/4 tsp freshly ground black pepper

Directions

1. If using red onion, place slices in a colander and run under warm water for about 10

seconds, tossing once, to remove harsh bite. Drain well.

2. In a large salad bowl toss together spinach, apples, pecans, feta, cranberries and optional bacon and red onion. Drizzle desired amount of dressing over salad and toss to evenly coat. Serve immediately after adding dressing.

3. For the dressing:

4. Add all ingredients to a medium mason jar. Cover with lid and shake to blend well (or alternately just blend well in a bowl with a whisk).

http://www.cookingclassy.com/apple-cranberry-pecan-spinach-salad-maple-cider-vinaigrette/

Chocolate Chia Pudding

Author: ifoodreal.com

I looooooooove chocolate. This satisfies all my chocolate cravings plus the chia seeds are filling and chock full of nutritious bad assery.

Yield: serves 1

Ingredients

- 3/4 cup almond (rice, soy, hemp, coconut, dairy) milk, unsweetened
- 2 tsp maple syrup/honey or 1/4 tsp stevia
- 1 tsp pure vanilla extract
- 3 - 4 tbsp chia seeds*
- 1 tbsp cocoa powder, unsweetened

Directions

1. Add all ingredients to a Mason jar or any container with a tight lid (I prefer glass) in the order listed above - liquids first. Whisk well or stir vigorously with a fork until cacao powder is well combined with the rest of ingredients. Refrigerate for at least 6 hours or overnight. When ready to eat, stir well again. Some lumps are OK, just stir well. The thickness and sweetness can be adjusted to your taste.
2. Storage Instructions: Refrigerate for up to 5 days.

Notes

* For a thick consistency pudding use 4 tbsp chia seeds, for soup like consistency (pictured) use only 3 tbsp (my favourite).

http://ifoodreal.com/chocolate-chia-pudding-recipe/

No Bake Oatmeal Energy Bites

Author: isavea2z.com

These are stupid addictive. I like to freeze them and eat them so the chocolate chips get crunchy. Crazy nutrient dense and great for the sweet tooth.

Yield: 18 to 20 bites

Ingredients

- 1 cup oatmeal
- ½ cup peanut butter (or other nut butter)
- ⅓ cup honey
- 1 cup coconut flakes
- ½ cup ground flaxseed
- ½ cup mini chocolate chips
- 1 tsp vanilla
- Optional: add dried fruits such as cranberries, blueberries etc...

Directions

1. Start with that gooey peanut butter, honey and some oatmeal and mix in a big bowl.
2. Then add in a cup of coconut flakes, sweetened or unsweetened…your call.
3. Then you can add in your mix-ins. I like to keep these somewhat healthy so I add mini chocolate chips and ground flaxseed. But you could also add in some chopped nuts, dates, raisins and even switch out the flaxseed to wheat bran or something similar or even cocoa powder. I love this recipe because it is

pretty customizable to what you have in your pantry.

4. Then add in a teaspoon (or two) of vanilla!
5. Mix it all up and let it chill in your refrigerator for about a half hour.
6. Then roll into balls and enjoy your little bites of heaven…or energy…depending on what you put in them!

http://www.isavea2z.com/oatmeal-energy-bites-bar-no-baking-required/

If you read through this little book and decide that you want to pursue this path and that you'd like some additional support, feedback, and accountability, please get in touch. I offer one on one coaching through my website and blog, www.jennicamaxfield.com/coaching .

Please feel free to get in touch with your comments and questions and share your successes with me so I can celebrate with you! Tag your photos with hashtag #easierthanyouthink to be sure I can find them. Here's where you can find me:

Website: www.jennicamaxfield.com
Facebook: www.facebook.com/jennicamaxfield/
Instagram: www.instagram.com/jennicamaxfield/
Twitter: www.twitter.com/jennicamaxfield
Other than that, everything looks good!